Optimal Fitness For Busy Professionals

How to be a Fit Corporate Professional, be More Productive, and Spend Less Time in the Gym.

By Nigel Lyons

DEDICATION

I dedicate this book to my parents Andy and May for giving me a good start in life.

Table of Contents

ACKNOWLEDGMENTS

I would like to thank my mentor, <u>Chris Lutz</u>, for all his help in the production of this book.

INTRODUCTION

"I don't have time to exercise! Fit exercise into my busy schedule? I'm already stressed out." These are the common things people say that stop them from exercising.

As we get older and have more responsibility, our career, home life and family start to get priority ahead of our own health and fitness.

While you can get away with this for a while, as you start to eat more and move less the pounds start to creep up, until one day you look in the mirror at yourself and realize just how much you've let yourself go. Worse, when you feel like you may have been conserving your energy by not exercising, becoming over fat and out of shape has led to a slower and more lethargic feeling in your daily life anyway. You haven't saved energy, you're more tired now than ever.

But it doesn't have to be this way. With a few simple changes to your lifestyle and a routine to keep you focused, you can get back on track. Something doable, practical, and sustainable for you. Not something outlandish that you'll never stick to. Something realistic and still can produce the desired results.

Maybe, you've never exercised before or engaged in any physical activity or you were once in good shape but life got in the way and you got out of the habit. A wife or husband, children and a busy career take over.

In other words, it's just not a priority. Unfortunately though, when we neglect ourselves, it starts to affect other areas of our life. If you have a stressful job then you need to be in good shape mentally and physically. Many people in corporate positions resemble athletes in a way. They have to moderate their efforts, conserve strength, and exert maximally when needed at ideal times. If you have 3 young kids then you're going to need some energy for them if you want to be a good parent. So many people give all of themselves all day at work and then come home to kids still running laps around the dining room table. They realize they now have three or four more hours of "work" to do at home before kids have finally settled and are in bed.

Companies are now demanding more than ever of their employees and sickness costs companies money.

In a report in Ireland done in 2009 entitled "Employee absenteeism- A guide to managing absence" it was found that absenteeism costs Irish businesses about €1.5 billion a year.

Business group IBEC claims that 11 million days are lost each year because employees take unplanned time off.

Also, for someone who is self employed and owns their own business, being sick generally means a loss of earnings or at least a reduction. This you cannot afford to happen consistently.

So we need to keep ourselves in good physical health and fitness if we want to have a productive career and lead a long, fulfilling life!

To start off we need to take stock of where we are at now. Have you really looked at your body lately? Have you taken stock of your overall physical well-being?

Before tackling the idea of fitting exercise into your busy schedule, it might be better if we start with the concepts of self-assessment and then familiarize ourselves with the disease-prevention aspect of exercise.

Once you've accepted the fact that your body needs overhauling, and that exercise is good for your health – then we can talk about some of the ways that you can include exercise into your roller-coaster existence.

This book in your hands right now (or on your screen!) is your KEY to fitting exercise into your life. And rest assured, this book already assumes that you're a busy person with a life to lead; and that's why the tips in here are **specifically designed to fit in with your busy lifestyle!**

To keep things organized and simple, this book is broken down into five easy sections:

Section 1: Assessing Physical Damage and Accepting the Importance of Exercise

Section 2: No Matter How Busy You are, There are Ways You Can Exercise

Section 3: Busy Traveler? You can Fit Exercise into Your Trips

Section 4: Exercise Equipment To Go

Section 5: Information / Resources

Read them in order, or if you wish, focus on the section that is most relevant to you right now. Regardless of how you choose to read this book, you can be confident of one thing: once you apply the advice within these pages, your busy life will include something new and important: exercise and a better you!

Myths and Misconceptions Surrounding Exercise

Before we get into the meat, lets dispel some of the common myths surrounding exercise and fitness. It won't do you any good to go into a health and fitness program with pre-conceived notions still lingering in your head. Let's wipe the slate clean and establish what is good and true information and what isn't.

To date, there are few industries with more misinformation than the health and fitness industry. It might be safe to say that for some of us, everything we think we know about it is wrong or misinformed.

"What gets us into trouble ain't what we don't know. It's what we know for sure that just ain't so."
– Mark Twain

Some of these are ingrained in people's minds because they heard it somewhere or read it in a magazine and just assumed it to be the truth, without any real thought behind the evidence supporting it or where it came from.

Read this book with an open mind and prepare to forget everything you think you know about exercise. With that said, here are some of the common myths:

Women will get bulky from lifting weights: This myth never seems to die! It is the irrational fear of every woman who picks up a dumbbell. However, It couldn't be further than the truth. Women do not have the genetics or testosterone levels to put on massive muscle. Hell, Its hard enough for the average guy to pack on some muscle! Strength training is the best thing a female can do to improve muscle shape and burn fat. It will enhance any feminine shape she already has. It will not make her shape appear more masculine.

You may see this in female bodybuilding, but that is because they are taking drugs that resemble male hormones which result in those characteristics. Things like facial hair are another side effect of those drugs. A normal and healthful resistance training program for women will do nothing like that. See more on the benefits of strength training in the next section.

You need to exercise for six days week to get good results: People also assume that if exercise is good, then more must be better right? Wrong! To get good results from an exercise program, all that's needed is training for three to four times per week with a good level of intensity. And It doesn't have to be for an hour either. 30-40 minutes should be plenty of time to give you a good workout over your whole body. Rest is equally as important as the work of exercise. Rest is when the positive adaptations actually occur to your body. We want to allow that to happen. The exercise's purpose is to set the process in motion.

Workouts too frequently can prevent proper amounts of rest and can contribute to overreaching or overtraining. People who do this often are forced to quit training due to their body's inability to handle the stress. You'll often see this inconsistency of a start and stop training regimen. If it isn't consistent, it isn't going to be successful. Allow for the right amounts of work and recovery.

Muscle turns into fat: People think if you exercise consistently for a period of time and then stop that muscle will simply turn into fat. This isn't the case. Muscle and fat are two different bodily tissues altogether and cannot transform.

This myth likely comes from formerly fit professional athletes who, having stopped competing, turn into out of shape people. This is especially true if they continue the same eating and consumption habits they are used to from when they were competing. You can see how this can quickly add up and they will add body fat without the constant demands of competitive professional sports. For us more regular people though, building a lean muscular frame will likely help us to raise metabolism in the short term and to hold off potential fat gain in the long run.

Running is the best cardiovascular exercise: Circuit resistance training is the best type of training you can for cardio. Moving quickly between exercises keeps the heart rate elevated for the entire workout resembling other forms of cardio. There may be slight dips in heart rate between exercises and spikes during the exercise resembling an interval which has been shown to be very effective for cardiovascular conditioning.

The cardiovascular benefit is the same or better as if you were jogging down the street except you are not exposing yourself to high forces that cause injury. You have to move your muscles to get a response from your heart. Your heart does not know if you are pushing on a leg press or running.

In a study more than twenty years old, a running and circuit weight training (RUN-CWT) program was compared to a circuit weight training (CWT) only program. In the conclusion of the study the authors state, "Statistically, one training program was not shown to be superior to the other; thus, both programs of RUN-CWT and CWT were effective in improving measures of physical fitness."

Does this mean that the running was just superfluous

activity? Possibly! Why wasn't the running and circuit training better? Your body cannot tell the difference between the two modes of activity. All it knows is that it is under stress so you better make sure that stress is safe and effective and not exposing you to *probable* injury.

Diets work: We're talking about fad diets here. Anything that is extreme in nature or programs that often demonize one food stuff over others. At any given moment, a large portion of people (especially women) are on one of these programs. They have been around for decades and yet, we're fatter than ever. What's worse, it might have actually caused us metabolic damage and trained us to be fatter than if we had done nothing at all.

Fat makes you fat: Simply consuming fat does not mean that it guarantees that it will be stored somewhere in your body. In fact, there are many types of fats, all have their purpose. Some are a critical component of your brain tissue and function and nervous system overall. Dietary fat can contribute to overfatness, but because of its caloric density. Fat is nine calories per gram vs. four for protein and carbohydrates. It's twice as dense calorically.

Carbohydrates make you fat: Carbohydrates are not as calorically dense as fat is, but they can play a role in metabolism as well as affecting the hormonal tone of the body contributing to an anabolic (storage) environment in the presence of too many calories overall. Too many carbohydrates can cause an eventual "crash" or drowsy or sleepy sensation sometime after consuming them. And can possibly contribute to a positive feedback loop in which you desire more calories from carbohydrate. All sugars are carbohydrates. But, not all carbohydrates are sugars.

Ultimately, they are broken down to their simpler forms and glucose is the primary sugar needed for energy production specifically for the muscular system and the nervous system. Too many carbohydrates can be converted by the liver into fat for storage. Fat cannot be converted back to carbohydrate for energy. Anything that supplies calories can make you fat, but carbohydrates alone don't equal fat gain unless consumed to excess.

Protein gives you energy: Protein does supply energy. Four calories per gram as noted above. However, it isn't the preferred source for some systems in the body like the nervous system which prefers carbohydrate. It is possible to survive in the absence of carbohydrates, but appears to be more of a last ditch effort for the body rather than the status quo. This is why someone can feel faint or dizzy with low blood sugar from not eating recently.

Fat and carbohydrate routinely provide the preferred fuels on a daily basis. You can think of proteins more for structural and metabolic processes rather than immediate energy. There is no storage place in the body for protein unless it is consumed with excessive calories and it can be stored as fat.

High protein diets make you lose weight: Although there can be a thermic effect from eating slightly more protein, the mere fact of consuming a *higher* amount or proportion of protein does not equal fat loss. Less total energy in calories than needed must still be consumed while taking advantage of the slightly higher thermic effect from a higher proportion of protein consumption. Protein, fat, and fiber can make you feel more full for longer and can contribute to less caloric intake overall with less discomfort from later hunger.

Aerobic activity (cardio) burns significant amounts of fat: It is true that the *proportion* of fat may be higher with longer duration and slower aerobic activity, but it is the activities or forms of exercise that are higher intensity that may require more calories overall even if the preferred source of fuel during that time is carbohydrate. It's really the deficit of total calories that determines the magnitude of fat loss, not the proportion of the fuel sources used in a given activity.

Aerobic exercise is safe: According to Dr. Ellington Darden, "More than 20 million injuries are sustained each year in the U.S. as a result of sports and fitness activities. To put this number in perspective, 20 million is more casualties than the people of our country have suffered in all our wars to date. Which activities are the most dangerous? There is an 86 percent probability of being injured each year if you play tackle football. That's self-evident because football is a combative sport. At 83 percent is gymnastics, which seems unjustified until you understand the very high forces involved and the great flexibility required to do many of the competitive events. Following at 80 percent is the popular aerobic activity, jogging or running. In the top ten is also aerobic dancing. At one time, in the high-impact years, aerobic dancing was at the 70 percent level of injury. Introducing the low-impact style lowered it to the mid-40 percent level. But with the arrival of step classes and the return of high-impact dancing, now called high-energy in many places, the numbers are moving back toward 70 percent".

Not only are these activities not safe, they are not necessary because the body's systems are so interconnected. It is not more effective or even desirable to break up training into strength and cardio or aerobics. It is entirely possible to combine the two for the most effect. According to Dr. Richard Lieber, "Since muscle represents about three-fourths of the body mass, a healthy muscular system is usually associated with healthy cardiovascular, pulmonary, and endocrine systems". Your muscular system is the one thing in your control (trainable) that you can use to elicit a desired response from your body as a whole for improvement.

Leg raises are for your abs: Leg raises are action around the hip joint. That means that it is actually hip muscles making the joint move. Specifically, they are called the hip flexor group. This is the primary group. People may feel some tension and burning in the abdominals during the performance of this exercise, but it can be confused with the hip flexors which run deep through the pelvis and abdominal area. Any abdominal action is secondary in this exercise. An exercise must flex your lumbar spine in order for it to be primarily an abdominal exercise. While we're at it, a six pack is not multiple muscles. It's only one, but is covered by tendonous inscriptions giving it that appearance. Nevertheless, it is only one muscle that pulls your chest closer to your hips. Functionally, that's about all it does besides helping to compress the abdominal space.

Spot reduction is possible: Nearly every mass marketed exercise device, particularly, abdominal exercises, relies upon perpetuating the falsehood that reducing fat in a particular area selectively (spot reduction) is possible. It simply isn't. Your body fat works as a system with our differing genetic make ups showing differing preferences for storage and loss.

You can easily see that this isn't true by the fact that overweight people who lose a significant amount frequently appear thinner in the face and neck. Obviously, facial exercise, although possible, isn't required to lose fat in that area. It won't speed it up either. It is stored in specific cells and used throughout your body as a system when required.

Warming up: Contrary to popular belief, a trainee's muscles will perform better if they are slightly cooler. Heat contributes to fatigue and ultimately heat sickness. We actually want to keep your body cool during a workout. Frequently, a warm up can be more dangerous than the exercise itself because of the high forces involved. Your first two or three sub maximal repetitions are the warm up. Sometimes a submaximal warm up set is used, but in general, it only takes a few seconds to bring your body temperature up to prepare for more intense work. Usually walking around for a couple of minutes after a workout is sufficient to prevent any negative post exercise effects.

Stretching: Stretching does not offer any protection from injury as previously thought. There is just now good research coming out that supports this. Most injuries are not caused by a lack of flexibility, but by trauma or too much force imposed on the systems. Stephen Thacker of the Centers for Disease Control (CDC) compiled a number of studies to look closely for any benefits that might be seen from stretching. Thacker says "We could not find a benefit." "And the injuries found in the study typically happened within the muscle's normal range of motion, so stretching them would not have made a difference."

However, this is not to say that it is never done. Generally, we want to design full range of motion exercises which includes emphasizing the stretching portion of the range. This is one way, but not the only way you can enhance flexibility through strength training. If desired, feel free to include a short stretching routine if you feel that it might prevent some later soreness and sometimes include 20 second stretches immediately after each exercise to stimulate a little more strength gain.

Some recent research has shown this to be possible. Other research has shown a slight correlation with stretching before activity and an *increased incidence* of injury so we usually stick to doing it afterwards if necessary. You should too.

Multiple sets: Conventional practice by most people is to use at least three sets and usually more. Statistically, there is little difference between one and three sets so only one *needs* to be performed taking other variables into consideration. However, over 96% of the research on this topic does not support or justify the idea that more sets are proportionately better assuming loads and intensity are the same.

According to Jack Wilmore, a prominent exercise physiologist and author of the book, Physiology of Sport and Exercise, "...it appears that a single set is just as effective as multiple sets for increasing muscle size and strength. In fact, of the studies that used appropriate controls, only one study demonstrated an advantage of multiple sets over a single set, and the magnitude of the difference in strength gains between three sets and one set was small." This being known and employed will result in an instant reduction of two thirds of the workout time. This alone should help convince some as to how it can be done in such a short amount of time which is perfect if you have a busy schedule.

Resistance exercise is dangerous: As noted above, some of the most common activities we use to improve our bodies end up hurting the majority of the participants. These are activities that are still thought of as safe even though the evidence would say otherwise. Although resistance exercise can be dangerous depending on how it is performed, it can be done in a very safe way despite the challenging nature and look of it. And despite added resistance to your musculoskeletal system, the total forces your body and tissues endure can be drastically less than repetitive , impactful, and/or forceful aerobic activities.

All is Not as it Seems

Now that we've established that nearly everything you thought you knew about exercise may or may not be true, let's go on to establishing where you're at now and getting you on the road to a better you the best way possible.

SECTION 1: ASSESSING PHYSICAL DAMAGE AND ACCEPTING THE IMPORTANCE OF EXERCISE

Do you think of your body the way you think of your car? When something goes wrong with our car or the oil light comes on we go straight to the garage to get it checked out. Better yet, we do preventive things to maintain it ahead of time *before* something goes wrong. We recognize that it's a large investment. We even insure our vehicles so that they will be around when we need them.

But when it comes to looking after ourselves we often take less care. We do far less preventive maintenance. We do insure our health, but you can sometimes never restore your body like you can a car after an accident. Our bodies are our daily vehicles that we cannot escape. It is our responsibility to do everything we can to function optimally and live a healthy life of longevity.

When we start to get the warning signals like high blood pressure, overweight we're slow to seek help or we will go to the nearest doctor to get some drug which may only masks the problem. And may even create new ones.

Shouldn't that person, shouldn't **you**, be the #1 priority?

Lifespan and Physical Appearance

The average life span of men and women is almost 80 years in the civilized world, give or take a few years. The painful truth is, a *significant* number of men and women look and feel 80 before they even make it to the first half of their life! You spot the tell-tale signs from their physical appearance:

- Sagging dry skin
- Unsightly posture
- Uneven and unsteady walk (they need to drag around those heavy pounds)
- Aching joints
- Sporting the "I'm not happy because I look terrible" look

Now, if their appearance is *this* bad, imagine what the body on the inside is like! Most likely, it's even worse:

- Clogged vessels
- Inefficient heart
- *Mounds* of fat parked in or around vital organs
- Conditions such as diabetes, high blood pressure and cardiovascular disease that are silently brewing.

Ideally, fitness would like to see exercise being taught from an early age, not during the teenage years when obesity is likely to strike.

But, fitness shouldn't be associated with any age limit. You can start at 10 or at 30 – even at 50 and 60 – the idea being that fitness should not be seen as the cure for a condition that's already come about although it can certainly be useful in reversing or managing conditions. As the saying goes, don't wait for illness to strike. Work with prevention in mind rather than cure.

Assessing How Fit You Are

It's important to begin by assessing how fit you are at the moment.

The following are some questions to ask yourself informally:

Start with the question, "**How do I look**?" Do any of these answers apply to you?

- Am I overweight?
- Do I have excess body fat around my waist?
- Do I avoid looking at myself in the mirror?

Next, ask: "**How do I feel**?"

- Do my joints hurt before or after any physical exertion?
- Do I get tired and lethargic a lot of the time?
- Do I suffer from mood swings?

Last question, "**How am I doing**?"

Are simple walking and climbing stairs difficult?

- Do I have problems concentrating?
- Is running impossible for me now?
- Are previously simple things a challenge now?
- Am I unable to sit straight, preferring to slouch or slump my shoulders?
- When was the last time I exercised?

You've completed your basic assessment. Note, however, that other exercise or fitness authorities will have their own parameters or indices for assessing your body's overall state and one isn't better than the other.

Physical assessments such as body fat percentage and

circumference measurements will also give you a good idea where you are at the moment in addition to just your total scale weight.

If you can, try to get these done from a qualified trainer.

For a more detailed look at where you are, you can use some **simple online tools to assess your current fitness level. Try this free fitness assessment.**

http://www.spartatraining.com/fitness-assessment.php

After going through the assessment phase, you're probably experiencing what some people call a "rude awakening".

The first step is acknowledging where you are and putting a simple and sustainable plan in place to regain your body and your health.

Goal setting

Before you start anything it's important to sit down and have a think about what you want to achieve. This well help you stay focused on the task at hand. If you have some pen and paper jot these down somewhere you will see them.

Do you want to lose 10kg? Build strength? Run a marathon some day?

Also, ask yourself **WHY** you want to achieve your goals? What would it mean to you? Often, these reasons are emotional ones like feeling better in your clothes, being more attractive to the opposite sex, improving your self esteem.

Think ahead to the future, what would It feel like 6 months from now if you had the body you desire?

On the contrary, what if you don't do anything now to change yourself, how will you look and feel in 6 months?

Asking yourself these questions can help kick you into action.

There are a few ways you can break down your goals using the acronym **S.M.A.R.T**.

Specific

Your goal needs to be specific to you there is no use saying I want to tone up. What does tone up mean to you? What areas are you looking to improve? If you want to lose weight, how much exactly do you want to lose?

Measurable

How can you measure your progress? I suggest you get some circumference measurements on waist, hips, thighs, chest and arms in addition to your total body weight.

Also, if you can get body fat measured. A skinfold calipers is probably the best method for this.

Achievable

Your goal needs to be something that is achievable but also challenges you to move out of your comfort zone. Something outlandish and that you know is unlikely from the start will only cause you to fail and lose heart.

Realistic

There is no use saying I want to lose 10kg in a few weeks. A goal should be somewhat realistic. If you are trying to lose body fat then 1-2lbs per week is realistic. It depends on your body and how much you have to lose. Conversion: 1Kg = 2.2lbs.

Timeframe

When do you want to achieve this goal by? Do you have a wedding coming up in the near future? Some sporting competition? Something like this will help keep your mind focused on the end result. And don't stop there, break the longer time frame down in to smaller chunks so that you can see if you are on track along the way. It may be a 6 month goal, but give yourself monthly milestones to hit along the way. If your goal is to lose 30 lbs, It's not going to happen in one month, so small chunk it.

An Additional Word About Goal Setting

The problem with goal setting in fitness is that the payoff is so far removed from the work. It's easy for excitement about accomplishing something to wane. Many times, this results in people becoming inconsistent, falling off the wagon, and thinking themselves failures. This cycle may happen to the same person several times over reinforcing the feeling of being a failure.

Here's what to do. In fitness ventures, most people often set or have goals in their mind. The most successful people have one type of goal over another. There are two kinds of goals to consider.

1. **Outcome goals**
2. **Process goals**

Outcome goals are usually how you envision yourself at the end or at some point out in the future. It's long term. You won't know if what you're doing is successful until you get there. It's good to have this long term goal/vision in mind, but not depend on it for long term motivation, feedback, and excitement.

Process goals are much more short term and not so much about what you'll look like at the end. An example of this kind of goal is more like to complete three workouts a week. That's it. Almost with no regard for anything else. But, it's something we already know is good for us and produces results. I've done that work and organized this for you. We know it will work in the long term assuming you stick to the principles. You now have to focus on the process goal of getting three workouts in per week. The process, with minor adjustments along the way, will take you to the outcome. It gives you immediate feedback compared to a long term outcome goal.

Did you complete a workout today? Yep. Goal achieved! You feel good about it. You get the same feedback at the end of the week. It serves to continue your reinforcement and excitement about where you are going.

This is really about enjoying the process along the way. You may not enjoy the hard work while you're doing it, but it's about appreciating the process simply for what it is.

Don't cry over spilled milk! If you get off your plan, that's ok. If you consume more calories than you were intending, that's ok too. Don't throw everything out the window and give up. It's about conserving what you've built up. In this case, it might be a good accumulation of workouts or a good calorie deficit. It would be like walking with a glass of milk and you spill a little. Are you going to stand there and pour the rest of it out on the floor? Or are you going to try to conserve what you have left? The latter, right? It's crucial to see the situation in this light. Not that any one thing is going to make you out of shape or fat again.

It's very important to build in some rewards for your actions that you accomplish during the week. Saturday or Sunday is a good day to reward your efforts in the process. Most people think of food when rewarding fitness efforts. Like having ice cream on Saturday night. That's perfectly fine, but it doesn't necessarily have to be food. After all, a smoker quitting smoking doesn't reward themselves with another smoke. I'm not saying you have to quit any food, quite the contrary. But, focus on all the things you like. What things do you enjoy that you can use to reward yourself with after accomplishing your process goals daily and weekly. It might be a TV show, a movie, a trip somewhere, a class you want to take, a shopping trip.

I personally think if you can incorporate the reward with something that will continue to make you excited about the next day or week's process goals, you'll be even more successful.

For example, let's say you accomplish your goals for the week and you get yourself a new piece of workout gear over the weekend. Now Monday comes and you'll be just a little more excited to complete the process using your new reward item.

This is the ultimate. If you can tie each part together so that the next effort either the work or the reward feeds the next step, you'll be in exercise nirvana. Going from the reward back to the process goal is obviously the harder part and key in order to be consistent.

Many people like to try a lot of variety. If that's the case for you, set a limit for yourself. Don't allow yourself to try a new technique or routine until you've completed a consistent routine three times that week. Or six times in two weeks. Just another idea. You get the point. Get creative and find what drives you to the next step.

Mindset

Don't under estimate the importance of a positive mindset when it comes to achieving your goals.

A lot of people sabotage themselves because they simply

don't believe they can achieve their goals. Maybe you've tried to achieve something before and failed and so you give up before you even get started.

Don't let failure hold you back on achieving your goal. Instead, learn from it.

Try and get to the reason why you failed. Maybe through reading this book, you will discover that you weren't doing things optimally. Maybe you didn't have anyone to hold you accountable and so you just gave up.

A tip: Get someone to hold you accountable to your goal. If it's to go to the gym 3 times per week, get a friend to go along with you, or invest in a personal trainer. There's a reason why people who have accountability achieve their goals quicker!

Whatever the reason is, learn from it and start again. People who are successful in achieving their goals refuse to give up at the first hurdle.

Raise your standards for yourself. Demand more from yourself than anyone else could.

3 success Factors

Throughout my time working with clients, I've found 3 critical components to their success.

1. **Responsibility**
2. **Consistency**
3. **Accountability**

Responsibility

Responsibility is about taking responsibility for your own success. It's easy to blame outside factors for not achieving your goals. "I have a slow metabolism. I'm too busy. She has it easier than me." Sound familiar?

The reality is that where your body is right now is a result of the decisions and actions you have taken over the last few years.

So accept responsibility for where you are and realise that you are the only person who can change it.

Consistency

Did you ever go to the gym consistently for about 4 weeks and then got out of the habit and completely stopped. It happens to a lot of us and it's the difference between people who achieve their goals and the people who go from one diet to the next looking for the magic pill.

Consistency is really about being consistent with exercise and nutrition from week to week and month to month.
You don't have to be perfect all the time, but being consistent is better than being perfect but not sticking to anything long enough to see any real long term progress.

Accountability

As we mentioned above, accountability is important to have when it comes to achieving your goals. The people you spend most of your time with can also have a big impact on you. If you want to go to the gym on a Thursday night but your best friend wants to go get a pizza, that's going to make it harder for you.

Don't be afraid to tell your friends and family about your goals. They should support you.

I have copied my top 10 client success principles here. These are the 10 principles I get my clients to adhere to.
Client Success Principles

1. Personal responsibility

Take active responsibility in your success, because no-one else can do it for you.

2. Know your goals

Know what you want to achieve, why you want to achieve it and how you're going to get there.

3. Have a healthy balance

Be good 90% of the time. Don't restrict yourself. Realise you won't be perfect and don't beat yourself up if you have a bad day. Pick up and get back on track.

4. Train hard

Give each rep, each set and each session 100%. Hard work equals results.

5. Be honest

If you're struggling, tell us. If you don't understand something, ask. There's no such thing as a stupid question!

6. Follow the instructions, keep it simple

Don't reinvent the wheel. And don't get caught looking for quick fixes or magic pills; there are none.

7. Eat real food

Eat whole non-processed food 90% of the time, while minimising alcohol, processed foods and sugar.

8. Post workout nutrition

Combine healthy carbs with a post workout protein shake after exercise to promote recovery.

9. Sleep

7-8 hours per night. Go to bed early. Recovery is the 3rd pillar of health, along with Nutrition and Exercise.

10. **Drink 2+ litres of water daily**

Over 70% of our body is water and it's crucial for fat loss and overall health.

Benefits of Exercise

If you make exercise part of your day, you'll experience some noticeable benefits. These include:

- Waking up in the morning feeling refreshed
- Walking with a spring in your step.
- Having energy left at the end of the day
- Feeling more optimistic about recreation
- Being more productive at work.
- Sleeping more soundly at night

Reasons to Strength Train

While exercise in general is a good thing, we want to make sure we are using our time to do the most productive exercise possible. Resistance training offers many benefits to everybody no matter what your age or goal is.

So here is a list of 13 reasons why Strength Training should be your exercise of choice taken from Wayne Wescott, Ph.D. and fitness researcher:

- **"Avoid Muscle Loss:** Adults who don't strength train lose between 5-7 pounds of muscle every decade. Although endurance exercise improves our cardiovascular fitness, it does not prevent the loss of muscle tissue. Only strength exercise maintains our muscle mass and strength throughout our mid-life and senior years.

- **Avoid Metabolic Rate Reduction:** Because muscle is very active tissue, muscle loss is accompanied by a reduction in our resting metabolism. Information from Tufts University indicates that the average adult experiences a 2-5 percent reduction in metabolic rate during every decade of life. Because regular strength exercise prevents muscle loss, it also prevents the accompanying decrease in resting metabolic rate.

- **Increase Metabolic Rate:** Research from Tufts University and the University of Maryland reveals that adding three pounds of muscle increases our resting metabolic rate by seven percent, and our daily calorie requirements by 15 percent. At rest, a pound of muscle requires about 35 calories per day for tissue maintenance. During exercise, muscle energy utilization increases dramatically. Adults who replace muscle through sensible strength exercise use more calories all day long, thereby reducing the likelihood of fat accumulation.

- **Reduce Body Fat**: Campbell and his co-workers at Tufts found that strength exercise produced four pounds of fat loss after three months of training, even though the subjects were eating 15 percent more calories per day. That is, a basic strength-training program resulted in 3 pounds more lean weight, 4 pounds less fat weight and 370 more calories per day food intake.

- **Reduce Resting Blood Pressure:** Strength training alone has been shown to significantly reduce resting blood pressure. Our YMCA studies have revealed that strength plus aerobic exercise is highly effective for improving blood pressure readings. After two months of combined exercise (Nautilus and treadmill walking), the program participants dropped their systolic blood pressure by 4 mm Hg. and their diastolic blood pressure by 3 mmh.

- **Increase Bone Mineral Density:** The effects of progressive resistance exercise are similar for muscle tissue and bone tissue. The same training stimulus that increases muscle proteins also increases bone proteins and mineral content. A University of Maryland study demonstrated significant increases in the bone mineral density of the femur bone (upper leg) after four months of strength exercise.

- **Improve Glucose Metabolism:** The University of Maryland research center has also reported a 23 percent increase in glucose utilization after four months of strength training. Because poor glucose metabolism is associated with adult onset diabetes, improved glucose metabolism is an important benefit of regular strength exercise.

- **Reduce Arthritic Pain:** According to a recent edition of the Tufts University Diet and Nutrition Letter, sensible strength training eases the pain of osteo and rheumatoid arthritis. This is good news, because most men and women who suffer from arthritic pain need strength exercise to develop stronger muscles, bones and connective tissue to improve joint function.

- **Reduce Low back Pain:** Many people suffer from low back pain at some point in their life. Several years of research on strength training and back pain conducted at the University of Florida Medical School has shown that strong low-back muscles are less likely to be injured low-back muscles. A recent study by at the University of Florida found that low-back patients had significantly less back pain after 10 weeks of specific (full-range) strength exercise for the lumbar spine muscles.

Because 80 percent of all adults experience low back problems within their lifetime, it is advisable for all adults to properly strengthen their low back muscles."

So to summarise everybody can benefit from having strength training as part of their routine. Also, there is a myth that women will get bulky from lifting weights. This is simply not true as women do not have the testosterone needed to build a lot of muscle. It's hard enough for men to achieve a muscular physique!

Reference: Westcott, Wayne Ph.D., Specialized Strength Training, Researcher at the South Shore YMCA

SECTION 2: NO MATTER HOW BUSY YOU ARE, THERE ARE WAYS YOU *CAN* INCLUDE EXERCISE

Are you always 'too busy' to exercise? Rushing to meetings, rushing home to cook and spend time with the family, surely, Exercise is going to take up too much of your time...

Then, we need to make room and find a way to fit exercise into your lifestyle so you can be more productive at work, have more energy and make more money. It's no secret that the people who make money and are the most successful in the business world are physically fit as well as mentally strong.

What if you could commit to 3 times per week for 20-30 minutes. Wouldn't that be manageable? Sure sometimes life gets in the way but if you can get into the habit of exercising regularly, it will become a natural part of your routine.

Then when you don't go for a while you will start to 'miss it' and that energetic feeling you get after a good workout will motivate you to come back.

A Time Efficient Exercise Program

Below is a suggestion you could use for fitting exercise into your schedule. You don't need to spend hours in the gym to get a good workout, this is a myth. Doing too much at the one time can often be counter-productive. Once you workout with a good level of intensity, less is more when it comes to exercise.

If you exercise with a good level of intensity and train hard, then 3 times per week is more than enough to keep you in good physical condition.

If you don't have access to a gym at the moment see the section, "When there's no gym".

Strength training has multiple benefits as shown in first section and can give you a better body composition than just doing cardio alone. Training with weights will help increase your metabolism causing you to burn more calories at rest. For this reason strength training gives you the most bang for your buck than Cardio. In order to burn 500 calories you would need to run on the treadmill for close to an hour. This is better achieved by just eating less calories in the first place!

Suggestion

30 minute total body workout three times per week e.g.

Monday, Wednesday and Friday. Your body needs some rest days in order to adapt and change. If you do exercise two days in a row then try to split it up into lower body/upper body so you won't be working the same muscles twice.

Terms

Before we get started with the details of routines, let's go over some terminology. *Physical activity* is defined as any form of movement. This could be a healthful experience or it could be a harmful one. There's no consideration for anything, other than movement here. *Exercise*, on the other hand is defined as a planned, structured, and progressive process by which significant physical exertion is applied to stimulate a specific desired and positive bodily change. A *repetition* is one single lifting and lowering motion of a resistance in any given exercise. It could also be a singular application of effort such as in the case of a static technique or a negative only rep which is just the lowering phase. A *set* is a group of repetitions performed together. The *positive* is the lifting of the resistance. The *negative* is the lowing of the resistance regardless of what the bar or body is doing. And there are different modes of exercise meaning the kind of exercise or the tool used. For example, a barbell bench press, the dumbbell bench press, and machine chest press are the same exercise using three different modes.

Sample Workout Routine

This is a full body workout which will work all the major musculatures in the body. This can be done in the gym or the equivalent with bodyweight if you don't have access to equipment. See guidelines for sets/reps intensity.

Leg press
Leg curl
Lat pulldown
Chest press

Cable row
Shoulder press
Calf raise
Abdominal crunch
Back extension
Tricep extension

Exercise Instructions:

Leg Press

Enter the machine by sitting on the pad with your back supported. You should be able to adjust the seat so you are not to far away and have a good range of motion. Lifting the legs up to achieve a 90 degree angle in the knee joint. Select a resistance that allows for 15-20 repetitions. You should begin the positive over the course of two seconds without a sudden jerk at the weight continuing into the upper turnaround without a pause. Make sure not to lock out the knees on this exercise. After a smooth upper turnaround, commence the lowering part for 4 seconds bringing the resistance down and proceeding to push just before the weight comes all the way down. Breathe continuously.

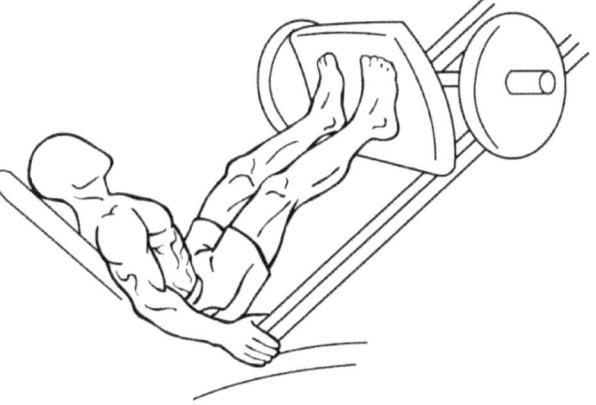

Leg Curl

These machines can come in either form seated or lying down in a prone position. Sit on machine with back against padded back support.
Place back of lower leg on top of padded lever. Secure lap pad against thigh just above knees. Grasp handles on lap support. Using your legs bend to fully contracted 90 degrees position. Pause for a brief moment squeezing the back of your legs and slowly return to extended.

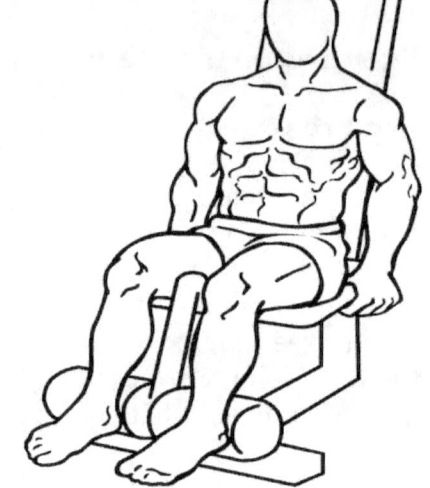

Pulldown

Begin by entering the machine by grabbing hold of the bar in an underhand fashion about shoulder width. Sit down while pulling the bar part way down. Lock the thighs under the thigh restraint pads. You should pull the resistance toward the top of the sternum or bottom of the neck and pause and squeeze after a couple of submaximal reps.

Proceed through the negative over 4 seconds under control and while depressing the shoulders and extending the elbows to maintain tension on the latissimus muscles. Try not to lock out elbow completely, and with smooth turn around perform the next positive. The scapula should rotate upward and downward,

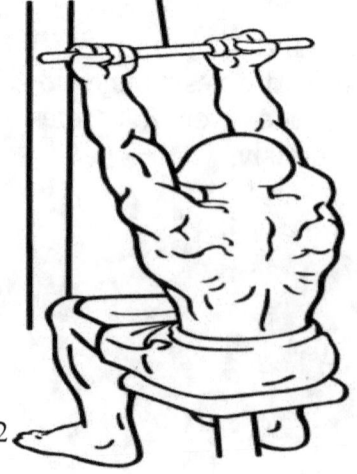

32

but the shoulder girdle should not elevate. To exit the machine, extend your elbows and slowly stand to set the weight down.

Chest Press

Adjust the machine so that you are sitting with the bars at chest height. Place your hands on the bars and place your feet on the foot rest. Press out, extending your arms but keeping a slight bend in the elbows before lockout and then return slowly to starting position.

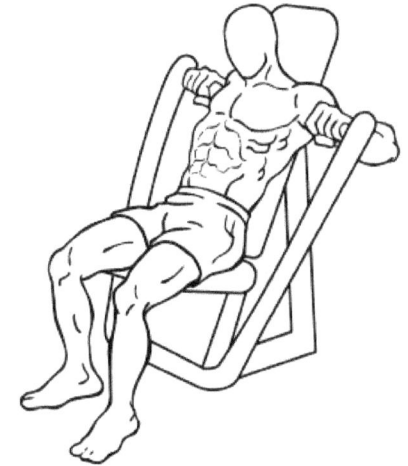

Compound Row

This is a cable apparatus, but the machine version can be used as well. Sit at a low pulley machine with your feet resting against the footrests and your knees slightly bent. With your abs drawn in and your back straight lean forward slightly to grasp the pulleys with an overhand grip (palms face downwards).

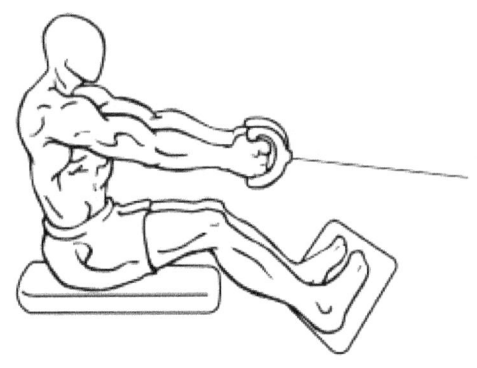

Slowly bring the pulleys back towards your abs while sitting upright, keeping chest high and your your elbows in close to your sides. Pause for a moment then return slowly return the pulleys to the starting position. Shoot for a two second cadence on the pulling part and four on the lowering.

Shoulder Press

Sit upright with your back supported by the chair and draw your abs in. Place your hands on the bars and with smooth even motions press upward extending your arms, but not locking them. At the top slowly start to lower with controlled motion back to the starting position.

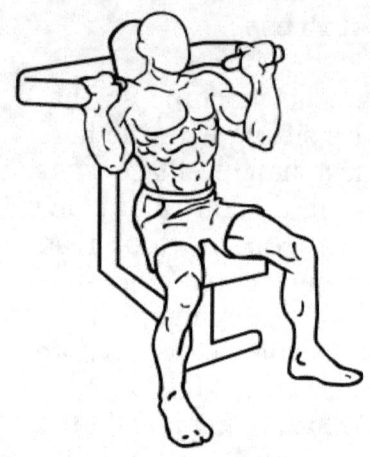

Calf raise

Most gyms have specific machines for this but they can also be performed holding two dumbbells either side and simply lifting your heels off the ground to come on the ball top of your foot and lowering back down. Also, something to stand on to elevate the feet will help give greater range of motion.

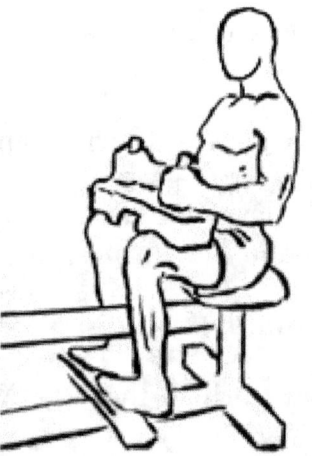

Abdominal Crunch

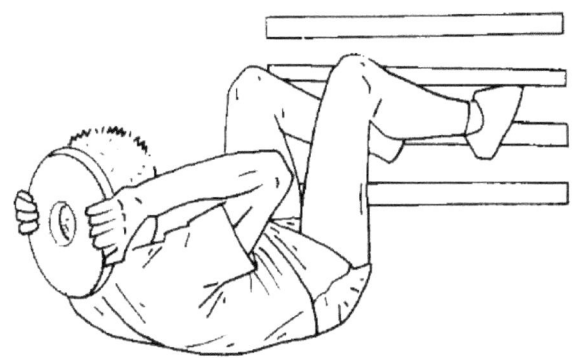

You can start by lying on the ground or a pad and feet propped up on a bench or stable surface so that hips and knees are bent at or near 90 degrees. Cross arms over chest or place hands behind head. Be careful not to pull on the neck during the crunch. Slowly commence a crunching motion tightening the abdominal wall muscles to flex the spine. You'll feel your lower back press into the floor. Think about bringing your chest closer to your pelvis. Pause and squeeze your abdominal muscles as tight as you can for a second and begin to descend in four seconds. Come down only until you shoulder blades just touch the floor, but don't let tension come completely off of your abdominal muscles. Try to keep them tense with your body weight or additional weight all the way up and down in the exercise. The exercise can be made progressive by holding a dumbbell or weight plate over your chest or behind the head.

Back Extension

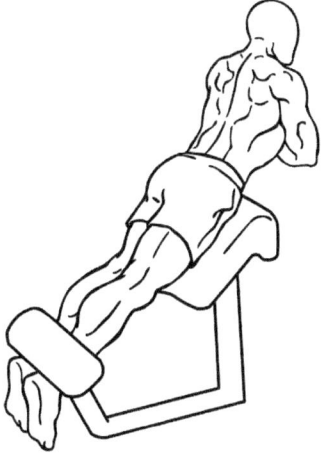

Be careful on this one if you have any pre-existing back condition. Position the foot pedestal high enough that you can safely climb in and position your hips just over the edge of the bench. When you gradually begin the positive, your hips and back should extend while maintaining a flat foot and slightly bent knee. You should exaggerate the extending motion pushing your chest up. Pause and squeeze in the contracted position after a couple submaximal reps then commence the negative taking 4 seconds to lower the weight. Lightly bottom out the resistance and start again. The back pad is aligned properly if it does not roll up and down your back during the excursion.

Tricep Pushdown

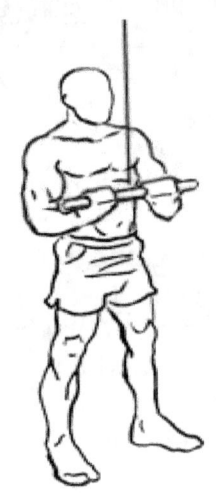

You should stand so that the elbow does not move forward as the negative is performed. Again, the positive is when the weight is going up, not what the body is doing. At the top of the movement, you can pause for a second and perform a squeeze technique for the triceps. You should perform slow controlled reps in a 2/4 cadence to fatigue.

*Images taken from www.everkinetic.com
Licence:
http://creativecommons.org/licenses/by-sa/3.0/legalcode

Specialised Routines

If you decide to train on two consecutive days, it's a good idea to break up the workout into a lower body/ upper body split.

These routines utilize the advanced technique of pre-post exhaustion explained below in "adding variety".

Lower Body

Leg Extension
Leg press
Leg Curl
Romanian Deadlift
Barbell/DB Squat
Seated calf Raise
Ab Crunch
Back Extension

Upper Body

Chest Fly
Chest Press
Seated Row
Biceps curl
Lateral Raise
Shoulder Press
Tricep Pushdown
Dips
Lat Pulldown

Three Day Workout Split

This is a 3 day split where you will train legs one day, chest, shoulders and triceps another day and then back and biceps. It's arranged in a leg, push, pull fashion. Follow the guidelines below or add one or two advanced techniques if you want an extra challenge. Be careful with your technique on exercises like deadlift and squats. If you need help get a qualified trainer to show you.

Lower Body

Leg Press
Leg Extension
Barbell Deadlift
Lying leg Curl

Standing Calf raise
Walking lunge

Push Day (Chest, Shoulders, Triceps)

Pec Fly
Dumbbell decline chest press
Barbell bench press
Lateral Raise
Machine shoulder press
Triceps Extension
Dips

I haven't included all exercise demo's here for a full library with demonstrations of the exercises have a look at www.everkinetic.com.

Guidelines:

Warm Up

For your warm up complete one set of a lower body exercise, and two upper body exercises, one pushing exercise and one pulling like a cable row. Select a lighter resistance (about 50% of what you would normally lift) and do 12 repetitions on each to get the blood flowing and your muscles warm. It isn't recommended to stretch before you start exercising. Some newer information is showing that it isn't a protector against injury and it isn't a warm up. Some has even show a slight tendency to more injury for those who choose to stretch prior to exercise. If you're going to include it, it is probably best saved for after the workout.

Reps

This is how many repetitions you do of each exercise. For the lower body exercises shoot for 15-20 reps and upper body 8-12 reps. The legs are a big muscles and can take a little more volume. If your goal is to build muscle you can lower the reps to 6-8 for upper body and 8-12 for lower body.

These numbers are just a guide. If you get to 12 reps and can do more then try to complete as many as you can. What matters is that your giving the body a stress that it needs to adapt to and respond during your rest periods.

Sets

To maximize efficiency perform 1-2 sets per exercise. The first set may be more of a warm up and your second set can be more challenging. Or what we call the working set. Where you can try to perform as many reps as you can in good form. Most of the research says that performing one set to a point of muscular fatigue (the point at which no more reps can be performed in good form) is just as good as performing multiple sets of the exercise. Be sure to have a spotter or equipment if you work to this point that will allow you to do it safely and not get pinned under any resistance.

Rest

Try to rest as little as possible in between exercises in order to maintain an elevated heart rate for cardiovascular conditioning as well. Strive for no longer than 30 seconds. If someone is on an exercise machine, it's ok to change your order and go to another exercise in your workout and come back. It's also ok to substitute the mode of an exercise. For example, if the shoulder press machine is taken for some time, it's ok to go over and perform a dumbbell shoulder press that day, just be sure to note this on your progress chart.

Breathing

It's important to breathe continuously through the exercises. If you find it hard, remember to breathe out as you lift the weight and inhale as you lower. Holding your breath during exertion can be dangerous. Forcefully building up pressure in your chest and abdominal cavity against a closed throat is called the Val Salva maneuver. And in extreme cases can cause stroke. Be certain to maintain an open air way and allow your breathing to increase in frequency as the exercise becomes more difficult.

Resistance

This will depend on your level and starting strength. You can start off low and then gradually build up. Because you're only doing 1-2 sets, you want the second set to be a weight that would cause you to reach muscular fatigue in the appropriate rep range (8-12). You can and should increase the weight as your strength improves. If you started with 5-pound weights, graduate into 7.5 pounds when you can perform 12 reps in good form. Try to increase your reps and/or weight each time you workout. This method is called double progression and it will serve you well in progressing over the long term. Anytime you can do up to 20 reps on any exercise with not much effort, increase the weight. Record your progress using a chart like the one below.

Example of double progression:

REP RANGE	WORKOUT #1	WORKOUT #2	WORKOUT #3	WORKOUT #4
8-12	150/11	150/12	155/8	155/9

Tempo

How you lift the weight is generally more important than how much the weight is. Everything should be done with a slow, controlled deliberate movement with no stop −starts unless you are performing a squeeze technique. You should take 2 seconds to perform the lifting phase and take 4 seconds on the lowering phase, this will minimise the risk of injury and make sure you are using your muscles to lift the weight and not momentum. You will see people move a lot faster than this, but they are most likely using too much weight and going too fast, a common cause of injury. Count the seconds as you lift to yourself if you need to, but after some practice you can get a feel for what appropriate speed of motion is without excess momentum or force.

Frequency

Three times a week should be optimal for most people. This will allow your body enough rest to adapt and recover from the workout. When you get more advanced, you may need to do less training to get the same results. Remember, more is not necessarily better.

Be realistic with your goals, especially when you're just starting. Increasing frequency too soon can overwhelm you, making you want to give up.

Intensity

Intensity is often lacking from most peoples workouts. Go in focused on giving every exercise and each rep 100% effort. A trainer or workout partner will help to push you. Exercise intensity should increase as you get more comfortable. Training to muscular failure is 100% intensity and requires concentration and focus while pushing past some degree of muscle soreness. Try to do better than you did in your last workout.

You can moderate intensity as time goes on. If you are exercising at a high intensity continuously and feel you need a break, don't be afraid to take a week where you lift lighter weights and give your body a rest. Above all, listen to your body.

Using RPE to Determine Exercise Intensity

Theoretically, all of the above would appear to be correct. In actual experience and for practicality's sake, not every trainee is going to train to 100% effort momentary muscular fatigue all the time. Beginners need some time learning the techniques with little fatigue at first. Other people may not have the same tolerance for high intensity effort output. And very advanced people may get to a point where 100% intensity in a longer duration set might actually be detrimental. The only thing we can truly know and measure is 0% intensity. Even a supposed 100% intensity will be rather subjective for a lot of people.

The scale we can use to determine your intensity levels is called the rating of perceived exertion (RPE). The original scale was a 6-20 scale held up in front of the trainee, usually while on a treadmill or bike, with different qualifiers for each level. 6-20 is rather hard to wrap your mind around especially while in a state of fatigue. Since we have reduced the scale to a simple 1-10 which many people are already familiar with and can easily comprehend. I'd suggest a 1-10 scale using qualifiers for the different levels like the following:

Traditional RPE Scale (1-10)
0. Rest
1. Very, very easy
2. Easy
3. Moderate
4. Somewhat hard
5. Hard
6. XXX
7. Very hard
8. XXX
9. XXX
10. Maximal

Now let's take that table and modify it or standardize it a little more specifically for resistance training. Obviously, terms like easy, hard, very hard are still extremely subjective and don't take into account any advanced techniques we might employ.

Resistance Training Specific RPE Scale (0-10)

0. Rest-No exercise at all
1. Very, very easy-Lifting movement arm or bar with no resistance on it
2. Easy-approx. 10-30% of 1-RM. 20-30+ repetitions possible at 2/4 pace.
3. Moderate-approx. 30-40% 1-RM.
4. Somewhat hard-approx. 50-60% 1-RM.
5. Moderately hard-approx. 60-70% of 1-RM.
6. Hard-approx. 70-80% of 1-RM.
7. Very hard-approx. 80-90% of 1-RM. 8-12 repetitions possible at 2/4 pace
8. Very hard-90%+ of 1-RM. Voluntary muscular fatigue followed by 1 advanced technique.
9. Extremely hard-possibly 100% of 1-RM+ (negative only, static holds) followed by an additional advanced technique.
10. Maximal. Voluntary positive muscular fatigue followed by 2 or more advanced techniques. Possibly reaching static and negative fatigue as well.

Without subjecting yourself to frequent max out attempts to determine 1-RM, use the following formula to obtain a predicted 1-RM.

Predicted 1RM= Weight Lifted(in pounds) / (1.0278 - .0278X)
where X = the number of reps performed.

Cardio

There's a lot of confusion about cardiovascular exercise. Cardio and weight training don't have to be two separate things. You don't need to be on a treadmill or cross trainer to work your heart and lungs.

Performing circuit resistance training with little rest in between exercises and training to fatigue will work your cardiovascular system simultaneously.

Unless you are training for a marathon or triathlon, you don't need to do long bouts of steady state activity on the treadmill or cross trainer. Research shows that shorter high intensity cardio is better for fat burning and body composition. So if you want to add some cardio then try something like this:

This would ideally be done outside in a park or a hill with a stopwatch or interval timer, but can be done on a treadmill. Spend five minutes warming up with a light jog, then for 30 seconds try to sprint at your maximal pace, take 60 seconds rest, then repeat for a total of 5 times.

When you're done your heart rate should be elevated and you shouldn't feel like you can do much more.

Depending on your fitness level you can take longer or shorter rest periods in between. Someone with a lower base level of fitness might need 60 -90 seconds rest.

These intervals can be useful at the end of your workout to increase your calorie burning post workout. Doing this prior to your resistance training will likely give you subpar results as you won't be able to generate nearly as much force during lower body exercises. In order to get the most bang for your buck, I'd recommend a resistance training circuit first and then follow it with intervals if you choose.

Resistance training is multi-dimensional in that it will address more than one component of fitness at a time. It has a contribution to cardiovascular, flexibility, and muscular fitness all in one. Cardiovascular exercise is more one dimensional. It doesn't really have a contribution to muscular fitness or flexibility.

Adding Variety

Another way to keep you exercising and motivated is to vary the exercise routine.

Variety promotes interest in maintaining your workout schedule. You don't necessarily have to change all the exercises but there are different ways you can manipulate the intensity to make sure you don't stagnate or plateau. Additionally, adding variety strategically can continue to stimulate improvement for the long term.

You could start to add more of the alternative equipment versions of the exercises as well. For example, your routine might call for the cable triceps pushdown, but you perform a dumbbell tricep extension. It's the same muscle, same action, and almost the same exercise. Chances are you'll be stimulating slightly different muscle fibers than using the same tool or mode of exercise all the time. But, again, don't just change just to change. You can go about it in a methodical way and still record progress your making in the short term with your changes. Ideally, only try to change one variable at a time so you can see what is really causing improvement.

Free weights

You can also swap some of the exercises listed above for a free weight version using a barbell or dumbbell's. Both have advantages and disadvantages and it's good to build a base level of strength with machines before moving to free weights which can require more skill depending on the exercise. You have to stabilise and control the weight when using free-weights which may disperse the load rather than concentrate it on your target areas. With machines, however, it makes it easier to push to a point of fatigue, whereas exercises like bench press require the assistance of a spotter or someone to help you lift the weight if you reach fatigue unless you are using a rack system of some kind.

Here are some techniques you could use to progress your routine if you start to see a plateau in your results. Note that many of these are advanced techniques that can be extremely difficult to recover from if used too often or if you do too many of them. Be sure to use them sparingly and moderate appropriately for your specific rate of recovery.

Rest Pause

This technique can be accomplished by performing a normal set of consecutive repetitions to fatigue followed by a 10 second rest and resuming a few more reps to fatigue. Continue two or three times. This technique may allow for a few more productive reps with just enough rest time to allow fatigue causing metabolic waste to leave the local area. Sometimes it may be as few as one rep, other times you might squeeze out another three to five reps. Do as many good ones as you can. Repeat if desired.

Breakdowns

Breakdown training is another form of advanced training to stimulate further progress. It consists of using your regular training weight in a set to fatigue and then immediately reduce the resistance 20

30% and do a few more reps to fatigue. This can be done once or as many times as you choose. Usually three reducing "sets" are pretty taxing and effective for stimulating progress over and above normal.

Slow Training

Standard rep speed is a cadence of 2/4. Slower speeds or cadences make the exercise harder for the muscles to lift the same resistance adding a new stimulus possibly in spite of lower resistance levels. These can be cadences of 5/5, 10/10, as long as 30 seconds to 1 minute or any combination thereof. An example would be the performance of a 1 minute chin. Take 30 seconds to lift your body in the chin up and 30 seconds to come down. The same can be done for dips or any other exercise if equipment allows. Challenging to say the least even with just body weight if resistance increases are not an option.

Static Hold

With static hold training, you hold the weight statically for a period of time. With the pushing exercises (chest press and shoulder press), about two thirds of the way through the positive is a good position to hold and for pulling exercises about half way is good. You can normally use more weight on this one than normal. Try to hold for 30-60 seconds breathing continuously and slowly resist on the way down in a slow negative.

Pre-exhaustion/Post-exhaustion

Pre-exhaustion is one of the most used forms of advanced training. It is really an attempt to get through a weak link in a chain. Imagine for example doing a set of machine chest flies immediately followed by the chest press. You pre-exhausted the larger musculature (pectorals or chest) with the first exercise and followed it with a compound exercise that also uses the triceps which are still fresh to more thoroughly work the chest. In the bench or chest press alone, the triceps are the smaller muscles and are the weak link and this is a way around that. This principle can be applied to any group of muscles and even applied in reverse which is post-exhaustion. A pre-exhaustion arm routine is one of my favorites. That is where you work the smaller muscles (biceps and triceps) first and follow it with a compound pushing and pulling exercise. Example: Bicep curl immediately followed by Lat pulldown. Tricep extension immediately followed by chest press.

Negative Only

Negative only has been promoted as the best technique so far developed. Since you are about 40-60% stronger on any given negative movement, this technique, as the name implies, uses only the negative portion of the rep. The chin up or dip is an excellent exercise to use for this technique. Start by getting into the top position by standing on something and ease into the transfer of weight and then proceed to slowly lower yourself taking about 10 seconds to perform the negative. Your effort should gradually increase with each rep and your speed should get faster until you are pulling up, but gravity is pulling you down against your best effort. When you can no longer go slower than about four seconds coming down, that is considered sufficient fatigue. I've also used this technique with much success on push ups for those that cannot do one or very many dynamic push ups. Eventually, negative strength builds so much that positive push up repetitions or full chin ups can become possible.

Negative Accentuated

This technique must be performed on a machine with fused movement arms. Many machines have movement arms that are independent like Hammer Strength. The performance of this technique is to lift bilaterally (with 2 limbs) and lower with only one. Alternate limbs on the lowering phases. First lower with one side, lift with two limbs back out, then lower with the other side. It is a great way to perform something similar to negative only on your own without a partner. Alternate limbs descending on the negatives. It is a great technique and variable for biceps and triceps machines, but can be applied to any machine with a fused movement arm.

Partial Range of Motion Reps

Over the years, it seems two schools of thought have emerged. Earlier fitness experts suggested moving in a full range of motion from full stretch to full contraction. More recently, the idea has emerged that you may be able to overload your neuromuscular system to a greater degree by using heavier loads and a shorter range of motion in your strongest portion of the range. Because we do not yet know which is better, if either, this style of training involves the use of both of these techniques. And it is an opportunity to insert more variety anyway or work around injuries. Generally, a full range of motion is used on any one given exercise.

However, especially from a post-rehab point of view, a full range may not be desirable and possibly irritating to an otherwise already injured person. The positions of full stretch and full contraction are largely myths. Many muscles have multiple "heads" which requires the adjacent limbs to be in different positions to fully contract the different heads. We also believe that a majority of muscle fibers can be recruited in nearly any position provided effort is high enough although this remains to be seen scientifically. We are not concerned with just inroading, fatiguing muscles, or loading them heavily. We are concerned with **ALL** of those aspects and the improvements from quality exercise seem to be a mixture of them all to differing degrees. The science is still in its infancy regarding these factors and their interconnected roles they play. Thus, all of these techniques have their place in a long term program.

Stage Reps

Partial range of motion reps can be a great variable to manipulate. Ellington Darden has referred to this as stage reps. You can divide the movement into halves or even into three different training zones. It makes sense to train to fatigue first your "weakest" zone. For example, perform 8-12 reps in the top half of the bicep curl to fatigue, then immediately perform 8-12 in the lower half to fatigue. Sometimes, you may reach fatigue two or three times within the same "set" of stage reps. The technique can be applied to machines and is particularly effective in working around sticking points with barbell or cable exercises. Simply perform the stages and document your or your efforts on the progress chart. It is an interesting and different challenge.

High Repetition Sets

Sometimes for an added challenge and a different level of intensity, you could try high repetition sets using ranges in the 15, 20, or even 30 rep area. A 20 rep barbell squat is one of the most challenging things anyone can do in a brief amount of time. Of course, this is along the muscular endurance side of the spectrum, but might also help to develop a little more fatigue in those that might not have done so deeply with fewer reps or those that have a high percentage of slow twitch fibers and, therefore, have more endurance capacity.

Non-Consecutive Reps

Most of the time, we are striving for a set of consecutive repetitions. By consecutive, I mean, maintaining continuous muscular tension the whole time without respite at any point until muscular fatigue occurs. I have purposely avoided continuous tension with some surprising results too. It usually works well for those with poor motor control or skill or low tolerance. I have used several forms of this. One is to perform a whole rep and set the weight down just long enough to take a breath and go again. Fatigue still occurs in a reasonable amount of time, but may help with some of the burning sensation.

Physiologically, it might actually help to stave off some of the fatigue causing reactions and squeeze out another one or two productive reps. It's particularly effective on something like the leg extension or other exercises where it is not difficult to get started out of the bottom position from a dead stop.

1 ¼ Reps

This advanced technique is great for use on single joint exercises in general, but specifically for the arms and legs. It is simple really, they'll perform 1 whole positive, lower the bar ¼ of the way down, then squeeze back into the positive and contracted position then proceed down on a full negative. It's like doing a double squeeze technique. You'll probably need to lower the resistance a slight amount at first as they'll fatigue pretty quickly with this technique. Try it on leg curl, leg extension, bicep curl, and tricep extension.

Modified Squeeze Technique

One technique I like to employ especially for some beginners and sometimes on an area like the lower back is extending the time a client spends in the squeeze position on a single joint exercise. Although the lower back is not a single joint, per se, but the machinery we use operates like one. Instead of a 1 second pause and squeeze in the contracted position, you would have the client perform it for a longer amount of time say, 3 or 5 seconds. This can help the client in identifying the actual muscular structures that are supposed to be contracting and learning how to contract them better going forward in their training. They can learn the difference between simply pausing passively and actively squeezing in the contracted position. It can potentially add a little more effectiveness to the set. And in the case of the lower back, spending an extended time in that position, it can help make the client's back feel better by decompressing the discs. Be sure to adjust resistance levels if necessary as this will cause fatigue quite a bit quicker than the usual squeeze technique.

Isometronic

Isometronic was developed by Peary Rader, the Iron Man magazine founder. It is a series of isometric or static contractions performed in short range movements. Here, a power rack can come into good use again. There are varieties of ways to perform it, but the easiest way is to do something like a bicep curl. Set the pins so that you curl the bar up and touch to the pins, but you cannot go beyond them. Try to break right through the pins with a maximal static contraction for five to 10 seconds. Perform a given rep range (8-12) in that position if you wish, but you don't have to. Then you can move the pins up to the next hole and progress through the range of motion using the same format. An alternative way is to load the bar with enough resistance that you can just curl it up to touch the pin and hold for 5-10 seconds. Then progress through the range.

Multiple Planes of Motion and/or Hand Grips

There might be some benefit to using different planes or grip positions. Again, I have yet to see this definitively in scientific evidence, but it stands to reason that it can pay off. Here's how. We know that nothing is perfect, there are only trade offs. There will never be a perfect machine or exercise due to multiple muscle heads, joint shapes, limb lengths, speeds, and different hand grips required, etc. Like the supinated lat pulldown may be a better grip for bicep strength, but it pulls the humerus (upper arm bone) OUT of what might be considered the best line of pull for the latissimus. The pronated grip keeps the humerus bone more in the direct line of pull, but the bicep is in its weakest position. You see? It's only a trade off and you can't do both at the same time. Does it matter? Maybe not? Could it potentially matter in the long run? Sure. So here is a way to address the multiple functions. Actually there are more than one way, but this is one example. It is sort of along the same lines of reasoning as a breakdown technique which we do know from testing has been shown to be effective.

Let's take the lat pulldown example again. The pronated grip (overhand) is the weakest position, the neutral grip is the second strongest, and the supinated grip (underhand) is the strongest position. So, instead of using one grip and performing a breakdown in resistance used, I'll perform the "breakdown" using the different hand grips. In quick succession, I'll perform a pronated grip (weakest position) lat pulldown with X weight. Keeping the same resistance, I'll switch to the neutral grip (second strongest), but I'm in a stronger position now, then perform the last in the supinated grip with the strongest position. In all instances, I was using a progressively stronger grip or hand position, but resistance staying the same even though I was fatiguing from each "set". So you get the effect of a breakdown and possible benefit of different angles or stimulation of muscular attachments. The same can be done on something like a chest press. Start with the incline, move to flat, then finally perform decline in the weakest position. You can use an infinite number of planes or hand grips that you wish. Three should be sufficient for both.

Timed Static Contractions (TSC)

Although I don't believe this technique to be as effective, it still has its place and definitely is useful for the post-rehab or working with injuries. It is representative of original isometric training. This is different from a static hold whereby you are holding a specific amount of resistance. During TSC, they are just exerting against an immovable object. I like to use a method of graduated effort and intensity. I break the time frame up into 30 second blocks for a total of a minute and a half. The first 30 seconds is moderate effort, the second is about 90%, and the third is 100% all out effort. You can differ your time intervals however you wish. By the end of this, the effect should be pretty high, but maybe not as effective as other techniques. We can thank Charles Atlas for popularizing this technique, but it has probably been around for centuries.

Beware of Overtraining

All of these variables can be put to use during the lifespan of a trainee's program. A word of caution though, overtraining is easier to do than people think. Use advanced techniques sparingly. They are good to use, but be conscious and aware of your responses. Some general overtraining symptoms are:

- Trouble going to sleep
- Trouble waking up
- Overuse atrophy
- Lack of performance
- Irritability
- Depression
- Elevated resting heart rate
- Persistent soreness
- Decreased appetite
- Injuries
- Decreased immunity

Everyone is different, pay attention to what your body is trying to tell you. Be conscious and aware. Once a person delves into overtraining, it takes time to get out. Think of it like digging a hole, the deeper you go, the longer it takes to climb out. If you do find your yourself overtrained, as many people are, your best bet is a couple days to a week off. BE CAREFUL here, however, as you don't want to get out of your routine. Just take what you need and then get right back on plan.

Walk Before you Run

If you're an *absolute beginner*, you can start out with a lower intensity and see how your body responds first. You may get some muscle soreness the next day the first few times, then after your body will start to adapt.

See how your body responds after the first workout. I believe in training hard but there is no use in killing it in the first workout and then being sore for a few days afterwards you can hardly move!

You could also integrate your favorite sport (swimming, cycling or walking) during the week. After all, that's why we do this training and preventive maintenance, so that we can do and enjoy those things.

Time Management

Time is the main reason people give for not exercising in the first place. But it's about how you manage your time and finding ways to incorporate exercise into your schedule. If your schedule gets you up and running beginning at 9 in the morning until six in the evening, this day represents 9 hours. There are 24 hours a day and we're not recommending you get up at 2 in the morning to do your exercise.

But have you ever thought that if you get up at 8 to be ready for 9, maybe you can set your alarm clock an hour minutes earlier, using 30 minutes to engage in a physical activity? If you do this three times a week, that means you get 90 minutes that you can allocate for exercise.

One easy way to do this is to do your exercise in the morning at home before you leave the house. If you have a mat and some light resistance you can still get a good workout.

See the routine on bodyweight exercises on page 29.
If you have a treadmill at home then you can do some high intensity sprints.

Another time management tip: not only do busy managers have back-to-back meetings, they also have luncheon and dinner meetings to meet with clients. Assess each client. Do all of them really need to be wined and dined? Is an hour long meeting absolutely necessary? Can't a deal be negotiated on the phone? Meetings can take up a lot of your time. Try to look for ways to make your time on the job more efficient.

See how many meetings you can cancel or shorten, but not at

the expense of your livelihood, obviously. Then fit your fitness program into those slots that have been freed up.

How about this suggestion: Instead of going to lunch with clients every day of the week, why don't you schedule lunch meetings for say Tuesday and Thursday? This way you can incorporate a fitness routine for Monday, Wednesday, and Friday from 12:00 to 12:30 pm. And then replenish your body with a balanced lunch after that workout.

A quick exercise session in the local gym or a run in a park nearby will leave you feeling invigorated when you do go back to work, rather than getting that 3pm slump and going to the coffee machine.

You could also go to the gym after work if it suits you better. It's better to go immediately after work than go home first because then you get comfortable on the couch and end up leaving it until tomorrow which never comes.

When you need to take a break during the day getting outside for a quick walk and grabbing a healthy snack will help you stay productive.

Some people bring exercise equipment into their office like dumb bells or elastic bands – where there's a will there's a way! Look for solutions for ways to fit exercise in, not excuses!

Family Activities

If you have a family and children it's a great chance to get some additional physical activity too. Take the kids to the park and go running or cycling with them. Are they off to their swimming lessons or skating lessons? See if you can sign up in the adults section, or take a walk outside the recreational center while waiting for them.

Walk or Cycle, Don't Drive!

Try to park further away from the office so you have to walk for a bit. Or if it's not too far and weather permits, try cycling into work. Some companies offer incentives like tax saving for people who cycle to work.

Nutrition

In order for you to feel energized to workout, you need to fuel your body with the nutrients it needs. Make sure you're getting a balance of all three macronutrients protein, carbohydrates and fats.

Protein is crucial for growth and repair of your muscles and other structures. Carbohydrates will be your primary energy source, and we need good fats also to help protect the joints, be a crucial part of the nervous system, and act as a secondary source of energy.

Good sources of protein are chicken, turkey, eggs, fish, and lean cuts of red meat. Aim to get plenty of fruits and vegetables as your source of carbohydrates and stay away from any processed or refined carbs.

If your one of these people who struggle to get enough vegetables in your diet then a greens supplement is a great idea. This is one I have used before which has massive benefits for overall health, fat loss, digestion and energy levels; http://goo.gl/7H1hww

Having one serving of this is the equivalent of your 5 portions a day. Having tried different greens drinks most are hard to take but this one actually tastes good, easy to mix and you get the numerous benefits.

For fats, go for the good ones like coconut oil, olive oil, avocados, and nut and seed oils. Fats have 9 calories per gram, a little higher than Protein and Carbs which have 4 calories per gram.

Having these three together will help keep your blood sugar levels stable throughout the day and provide you with energy.

Having healthy snacks will prevent you from making bad choices and going to the nearest fast food restaurant.

Nuts, sesame seeds, protein bars, some dried and fresh fruit, baby carrots, cereal flakes, oatmeal bars should keep you on the go while exercising.

You could even make your own protein bars and have them for snacks when you're on the go. Here is a recipe you could use:

3-4 scoops Whey protein Powder, 1 ½ cup oats, 2 table spoons flaxseed, 2 tablespoons peanut or almond butter, half cup milk, handful of raisins, cinnamon, coconut flakes.
To prepare get all the ingredients and mix in a bowl.

When mixed, spread over and pat down on a baking tray lined with wax paper or tinfoil and sprayed with some oil to prevent sticking. Sprinkle the coconut over. Store in the freezer for 30-40 minutes or until hard.

When you take out you should be able to cut into 5-6 separate bars, then store in the fridge in tupper ware.

If you're pressed for time to sit down for a proper meal, these portable foods will hold you over in a healthy and nutritious way.

If you are trying to lose body fat it's important to get an idea of how many calories you need first. You can use a formula like the Harris Benedict one:

English BMR Formula

Women: BMR = 655 + (4.35 x weight in pounds) + (4.7 x height in inches) - (4.7 x age in years)

Men: BMR = 66 + (6.23 x weight in pounds) + (12.7 x height in inches) - (6.8 x age in year)

Metric BMR Formula

Women: BMR = 655 + (9.6 x weight in kilos) + (1.8 x height in cm) - (4.7 x age in years)

Men: BMR = 66 + (13.7 x weight in kilos) + (5 x height in cm) - (6.8 x age in years)

This number is how many calories you need just to function. Look at the following chart to factor in your activity levels:

Sedentary: Little to no regular exercise × 1.2

Mild activity level: Intensive exercise for at least 20 minutes 1-3 times per week × 1.375

Moderate activity level: Intensive exercise for at least 30-60 minutes 3-4 times per week × 1.5

So, BMR × activity level = How many calories you need to maintain your bodyweight.

If you want to lose weight you need to make sure you are in a calorie deficit. Which means the calories you burn is greater than the amount of calories you consume. Try not to depend on calorie "burn" from exercise. In fact, figuring as little activity into the equation is good so as to be conservative. You don't want to fall into the trap of over eating and then thinking "It's ok, I'll just burn it off later." In reality, it takes many, many times longer to burn off what takes a few seconds to eat.

A good guide is to take your number above and subtract 500. This is the an average of how many calories you should take in if you want to lose body fat.

There are 3,500 calories in 1lb of body fat. So if you create that 500 calorie deficit daily over seven days in a week, you should be losing 1 pound per week.

A good way to track your calories is to use the website www.myfitnesspal.com. They also have an app for smart phones which is very handy.

You don't have to continuously track everything you eat for months on end, but even doing so for three weeks will set you off on a new habit formed and make you much more aware of what is actually going in your body.
It's easy to under-estimate how much you're consuming!

Don't get too hung up on the scale body weight as this is not an accurate measurement of changes in body composition. See how you look and get a qualified trainer or friend to take circumference measurements like waist, hips, arms, thighs every four to six weeks to track your progress.

Lastly, we are all human. Some people have a sweet tooth like me. If you are good 80-90% of the time you can allow yourself some treats. Maybe take one day at the weekend to have something you have been craving. As long as you don't go to extremes, you will be fine.

Here is a reference list of over 7000 foods with nutritional info for each. To access this and download click here: http://wp.me/a33rSH-4u

The calorie tracker below will help you keep track of calories. Click on the image to download it in an Excel spreadsheet. You can do it the old fashioned way by printing it and filling it in by hand or keep it on your computer and fill it in there.

Calorie Tracker

Enter calories per meal for the corresponding day below. Replace the 1500 calorie day goal with your personal goal.

Start Date: _____

	Mon	Tue	Wed	Thu	Fri	Sat	Sun	Meal Notes:
Breakfast								_____
Snack 1								_____
Lunch								_____
Snack 2								_____
Dinner								_____
Day Total	0	0	0	0	0	0	0	
Day Goal	1500							
Difference	-1500	0	0	0	0	0	0	

Week Notes: _____

_____

_____

Sample Meal Plan

1500 Calories High Protein

Day 1
Breakfast
1 serving Louis Rich Turkey Bacon
1/4 cup Egg Whites
1 cup instant oatmeal, prepared w/ water
1/2 tsp ground cinnamon
1 cup orange juice

Lunch
1 Lean Cuisine Comfort Classics Honey
Mustard Chicken w/ Rice Pilaf
1/2 cup cooked green peas
1 tsp Benecol Light Spread
1 cup low fat milk, added protein

1 oz protein powder

Dinner
*1/3 cup Broccoli, Cheese, Rice Casserole
90 grams roasted turkey breast
1 whole wheat dinner roll
1 Tbsp Benecol Light Spread
1/2 cup strawberries
Snacks
120 grams low carb strawberries & cream yogurt
3 Tbsp ground flax seed

Day 2

Breakfast
1 serving Louis Rich Turkey Bacon
1/4 cup Egg Beaters
1 cup instant oatmeal, prepared w/ water
1/2 tsp ground cinnamon
1 cup orange juice

Lunch
1 Lean Cuisine Comfort Classics Honey
Mustard Chicken w/ Rice Pilaf
1/2 cup cooked green peas
1 tsp Benecol Light Spread
1 cup low fat milk, added protein
1 oz protein powder

Dinner
*1/3 cup Broccoli, Cheese, Rice Casserole
3 oz roasted turkey breast
1 whole wheat dinner roll
1 Tbsp Benecol Light Spread
1/2 cup strawberries

Snacks
4 oz low carb strawberries & cream yogurt
3 Tbsp ground flax seed

Day 3
Breakfast
1 banana
1 slice zucchini bread w/ nuts
12 fl oz low fat milk, added protein
1 1/2 oz protein powder

Lunch
2 slices whole wheat bread
1 slice low sodium Ham
28 grams low sodium cheddar cheese
1 tsp yellow mustard
1 leaf lettuce
1 slice red onion & 1 slice red tomato
2 celery stalks, 8"
2 Tbsp fat free ranch dressing

Dinner
100 grams roasted pork tenderloin
1 baked sweet potato
1 tsp ground cinnamon
1 cup cooked spinach
1 Tbsp Benecol Light Spread

Snacks
1 peach & 6 walnuts
1/5 cup low fat cottage cheese, no added Sodium

Day 4
Breakfast
1/4 cup Egg whites
14 grams low sodium cheddar cheese
1 cup low carb berries & cream yogurt
1/2 cup blueberries
1 cup low fat milk, added protein
28 grams protein powder

Lunch
4 1/2 oz Baked Spicy Fish
2/3 cup cooked brown rice
1 1/2 tsp Benecol Light Spread
1/2 cup honeydew

Dinner
450 grams Chicken Cacciatore Casserole
1 whole wheat dinner roll
1 tsp Benecol Light Spread
1 cup romaine lettuce
8 cherry tomatoes
1 1/2 Tbsp Italian dressing, no salt added

Snacks
1/3 cup hummus
10 baby carrots

Day 5
BREAKFAST
1/2 cinnamon raisin bagel
2 Tbsp unsalted peanut butter
1 cup strawberries
1 cup low fat milk, added protein
1 oz protein powder

LUNCH
1 wheat bun
2 oz Cripple Creek Pulled Pork
2 Tbsp low sodium barbecue sauce
1 apple

DINNER
*1 serving Crispy Cod Fillets
1/2 cup cooked cauliflower
1/2 cup cooked green beans
2 whole wheat dinner rolls
1 Tbsp Benecol Light Spread

SNACKS
4 oz low carb vanilla cream yogurt
1/4 Tbsp ground flax seed

Day 6
BREAKFAST
1/2 cup cantaloupe
1 oat bran muffin
1 Tbsp Benecol Light Spread
1 cup non fat plain yogurt
1 cup low fat milk, added protein
1 oz protein powder, 1 Tbsp fiber mix

LUNCH
1 whole wheat bun
1 Morningstar Farms Grillers Veggie Burger
2 oz low fat cheddar cheese
1 leaf lettuce
1 slice red onion & 1 slice red tomato
1 tsp yellow mustard
1 cup grapes

DINNER
2 oz roasted chicken breast
1 1/2 cup romaine lettuce
8 pecans
8 baby carrots & 5 cherry tomatoes
3 Tbsp calorie free Raspberry Vinaigrette

SNACKS

1 Protein bar

Day 7
Breakfast
2 oat bran waffles
1 serving Atkins Syrup, Sugar Free
1 tsp Benecol Light Spread
1 cup raspberries

1 cup low fat milk, added protein
1 oz protein powder

Lunch
2 slices whole wheat bread
3 oz roasted turkey breast
28 grams low sodium cheddar cheese
1 Tbsp light mayonnaise
28 grams unsalted soy nuts
1 cup watermelon

Dinner
1 Healthy Choice Familiar Favorites Tuna
Casserole Entrée
1 1/2 cup romaine lettuce
4 baby carrots
5 cherry tomatoes
1 1/2 Tbsp reduced ranch dressing

Snacks
4 oz low carb vanilla cream yogurt
1 Tbsp ground flax seed

This meal plan should be appropriate for most men and women. If you find from your calculations above that your metabolism is lower than this, then you can leave out one or two of the snacks throughout the day. This may be particularly true for some smaller framed women. Men have more muscle so metabolisms will generally be higher.

Nutrient Analysis

Nutrients	Day 1	Day 2	Day 3	Day 4	Day 5	Day 6	Day 7
kcals	1542	1509	1482	1510	1527	1559	1519
Protein (g)	119	114	116	130	113	122	123
Carbs (g)	175	169	168	152	171	181	157
Fats (g)	44	43	43	42	46	43	48
Cholesterol (mg)	130	153	149	200	144	81	156
Trans Fat (g)	0	0	0	0	0	0	0
Saturated Fat (g)	11	11	11	11	11	11	11
Fiber (g)	30	27	24	24	23	24	31
Sugar (g)	83	61	80	60	68	101	53

If the thought of tracking everything you eat initially scares you, you could try a more habit based approach.

Long term sustainable results with exercise and nutrition are suited best to habit building.

So, rather than completely overhauling your diet, you start with some little changes and progress as time goes on.

Not drinking much water? Then start off by drinking a litre of water a day? Then increase to 2 litres.

Lacking protein in your diet? Start off by incorporating a high protein breakfast such as eggs.

Are you currently taking an Omega 3 fish oil?

If not then start taking a fish oil every day.

For more ideas, have a look at my client success principles.

The idea is to start small and build on habits.

5 new habits done consistently over time will have massive impacts on your success.

People who say "Ok that's it, I'm giving up sugar and alcohol for the next few weeks" normally don't last too long before they go back to old habits.

If you drink a bottle of coke everyday then rather than trying to completely eliminate it drop it down to 2 a week.

The most important part of a diet is that you can adhere to it long term. If you can't stick to it, then it doesn't matter how good it is, it won't work.

Nutritional Supplements

With all the heavy marketing of supplement companies you'd be forgiven for thinking that you need lots of supplements to achieve your goals.

Really, there are only a few most people need to take. The most important part to get right first is your diet.

Supplements can help aid your diet and your health and

performance, but they can't replace a poor diet.

With that said, there are a few I take and would recommend to my clients.

1. A general multivitamin – This helps cover any deficiencies you may be lacking from your diet. There are good and bad multivitamins. Check out your local health store or go to **www.nigel.getprograde.com**

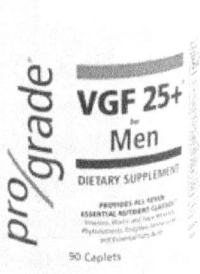

to get a high quality one.

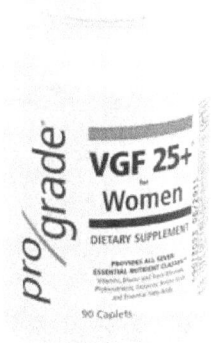

For men: http://nigel.getprograde.com/multi-vitamin-for-men.html

For women: http://nigel.getprograde.com/multivitamin-for-women.html

2. Omega 3 fish oil – there's numerous health benefits to taking a fish oil including joint health, brain function and metabolism. It can also help aid fat loss too. http://nigel.getprograde.com/essential-fatty-acid.html

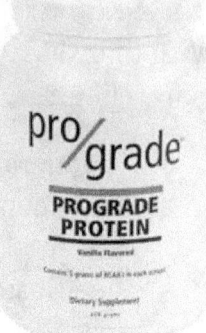

3. Whey Protein shake – For people who tend to lack protein in their diets, this can be a great option. It's also useful for post workout nutrition if you have a big gap in between your workout and your next meal. Look in your local health store or buy online here. http://nigel.getprograde.com/protein-powder.html

4. Although supplementation isn't a replacement for a poor diet, there are times where convenience can take precedence. If eating enough or at regular intervals is a weakness for you, consider a meal replacement. Many people skip breakfast entirely which can be a mistake. A meal replacement can be a simple fix to that problem. http://nigel.getprograde.com/meal-replacement.html

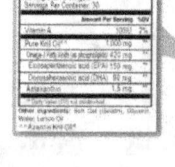
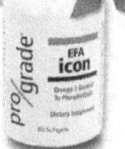

5. Creatine – Creatine is one supplement that's

being proven to help strength and muscle mass. I've supplemented on an off with this one and found great increases in strength.

6. Vitamin D – For people who live in less Sunnier climates (i.e Ireland)! Vitamin D can be useful and has a lot of health benefits.

Please check with your doctor before taking any supplements.

For un-biased research on supplements have a look at www.examine.com

SECTION 3: BUSY TRAVELER? YOU CAN FIT EXERCISE INTO YOUR TRIPS!

If you're a busy traveler who's always going from one plane to another, then it's easy

o to use that as an excuse not to exercise. But if you stay in any modern hotel there's bound to be a gym and even if there's not, we got you covered!

When you travel its easy to get run down going between different time zones, but a good exercise session will give you energy and make you feel better.

If you have a routine at home then you should be able to practice something similar in the gym the hotel provides but you can also switch it up and do something different.

Common Obstacles

What are some of the reasons why travelers do not incorporate exercise while they're on the road?

They're stressed or too tired. They don't feel comfortable about working out in unfamiliar surroundings. They don't have access to a hotel gym

But if they made just a tiny effort to change this thinking, they'd be on the road to fitness sooner. Engaging in exercise allows you to get out of that bubble of meetings, seminars and tours.

Walk when on the Road

When traveling, have a pair of good comfortable shoes (trainers preferably) so that you can walk comfortably from one end of the airport to the other!

Having comfortable footwear will encourage you to walk up the stairs instead of take the escalator, to walk instead of taking the conveyor belt, and to transfer from one concourse to another on foot instead of taking the shuttle service.

Also walking some distance with some suitcases is like walking with some dumbbells as resistance!

Fitness while Flying

Ideally you would be seated on the outside of an aisle so you can get up and walk about easily. If it's just an hour's flight, walk around the plane once and do some stretching at the back of the plane; if it's a three hour to five hour, try to get up from your seat and walk around at least once every hour, doing leg extensions and trunk/neck movements.

You could also do some body weight squats in the toilet to help improve blood flow to the legs. Just don't spend all day in there!

This will help make sure you're not too stiff when you get off the plane and help improve your overall mood and energy.

If you're going on longer flights crossing the Pacific or Atlantic oceans, you can increase the frequency of your stretches and walking.

Some airlines such as Japan airlines show videos of how travelers can incorporate flexibility movements while seated or standing. Take full advantage of these videos. The exercises may help you ward off fatigue and jet lag.

A Note about DVT

In the last five years, there have been reports about flight passengers, especially in economy class, suffering from DVT – deep vein thrombosis.

The link between confining airplane seats and deaths from DVT (formation of deadly blood clots) has been established by the United Nations World Health Organization. It has nothing to do with gender, risk factors or genetics. Everyone is at risk in economy class![1] This should constitute compelling reason to integrate exercise while high in the sky.

To make exercise possible while traveling, schedule your

flights so that when you get to your destination, you don't rush through dinner and then go to sleep.

Try to arrive during the late afternoon/early evening, to give you time to shake off the fatigue from the trip, and have at least an hour to do exercises either in your hotel room or in the hotel gym.

Important "to do" Things when Traveling

Be fully rested before a trip – have the usual "to pack" items ready well in advance so you're not scampering for them at the last minute, depleting your energy levels.
Time your sleep correctly – as soon as you board, get the local time of your destination and set your watch accordingly. If it's already night time in your destination, wear blindfolds and ask for a pillow and try to get some sleep. .

Drink plenty of water – wine and cocktails will only dehydrate you further; note that humidity levels inside aircraft is below 10%, so water is your best bet.

If your job requires you to travel at least four times a month, ask your company's travel department to book you in hotels with gyms or a swimming pool.

Make time out of your travel schedule to insert a workout into your grinding schedule.

Here's a friendly suggestion: get up earlier in the morning and before or after breakfast, head over to the gym and do a weight training routine for 20 minutes. You could do three exercises back to back: One leg exercise (Squat), one pushing exercise like a push up or chest press and one pulling like a lat pulldown. Perform 12 reps of each with little rest and try to do three rounds, resting no more than 30 seconds after each exercise. You can start with a higher resistance and decrease the weight after the first round. This session will wake you up for the day and should have you done in 10-20 minutes.

Now, tell us, doesn't a 10-30 minute session sound less intimidating than clocking 1.5 hours in the gym?

Working Out with Friends

Another friendly suggestion: If you're traveling in a group, ask a colleague if he or she would like to go to the gym with you. This can help motivate you and you can push each other and assist on some of the exercises.

When There's No Gym!

If you can't make it to the gym or you don't have access to one, it's not an excuse not to exercise! You can still exercise in the comfort of your room.

Here is a routine of exercises you can perform similar to the one in the gym but just using your bodyweight as resistance. If you have dumbbells, resistance bands or ankle weights you can progress some of these exercises. You could do these in a circuit like fashion doing 3 rounds for 12-15 reps. This will keep your heart rate up and as your not using resistance you can do a little more volume.

Exercise

Squats
Push ups (wide grip/Close grip)
Hip bridge
Lunges
Seated Band Row
Abdominal Crunch
Lateral Raise (dumbbells or resistance bands)
Back extension
Plank

Exercise instructions:

Squat

Feet hip distance apart, arms extended shoulder length, abdominals braced, bend the knees sitting your hips back squatting down till a 45-90 degree angle is achieved, keeping a neutral spine and making sure to keep your head up and not round the back.

This one can be practiced by sitting into a chair and standing back up. The knees stay tracking the toes. Keep the fleet flat.

Push Ups

Start with a basic push up, lay face down on the floor, or a mat; with your feet together curled slightly so you rise onto the ball of your feet. Place you hands shoulder width apart on the either side of your chest.

Inhale as you raise your body up till your arms are straight. Keep your head and neck level with your body (don't look up or down) and don't allow your back to rise or fall. Exhale out as you lower your body back to the ground.

Hip Bridge

This can be done lying down on a mat. Feet hip distance apart with feet flat and knees bent, hands rested either side. Pushing feet into the ground, you drive the hips upwards, pausing for a second and lowering back to starting position. This can also be done statically. Actively squeeze the hamstrings and glutes.

Variations: Hold statically at the top or bring hands over torso and elbows off the floor.

Lunges

Stand with feet hip distance and hands on hips. Lunge forward with first leg. Land on heel then forefoot. Lower body by flexing knee and hip of front leg to about 90 degrees, until knee of rear leg is almost in contact with floor. Return to original standing position by forcibly extending hip and knee of forward leg. Repeat by alternating lunge with opposite leg.

Seated Band Row

Sit on the floor with you legs extended and your knees slightly bent. Keep your back straight, wrap the resistance bands around your feet and hold each hand with your thumbs wrapped around the handles. Draw your arms back, keeping your arms close to your ribs, your elbows are in line with your back. Slowly lower back and then repeat.

Lateral Raise

With dumbbells or bands: Stand with feet hip distance and a slight bend in knee. Grasp handles in each arm, facing each other in front of your thighs, with a slight bend in the elbows. Raise the dumbbells slowly up to shoulder height, keeping arms relatively straight, then slowly lowering back down. If you can, try to pause for one second at the top.

Back Extension

Lying down flat on a mat, with legs extended and hands behind ears, lift your chest off the ground, then slowly lower back. Try not to strain your neck or do the movement too fast.

You can also progress bodyweight exercises through different ways. Here are some:

Squat

Perform statically. Bend the knees to about 90 degrees and try to hold that position for 20-30 seconds, keeping a neutral spine. (Challenging to say the least!)

Also, you could slow down the tempo of the exercise. This goes for all exercises mentioned above. Taking the squat as an example, If you lower down for 4 seconds, and proceed up for 2 seconds. This will make the exercise a lot harder than simply squatting up and down at a faster pace.

Push Ups

Try to perform the exercise is a slow and controlled manner. Lowering down for 4 seconds, and back up for 2 seconds.

Also, you could perform the exercise to fatigue, then try to complete some post fatigue negative reps. This is an advanced technique where you just do the lowering phase but try to draw it out for 5 seconds. Your eliminating the weaker part where you push yourself back up.

SECTION 4 : EXERCISE EQUIPMENT "TO GO"

You can generally use your bodyweight for a lot of exercises as above but if you want to progress it or change it up then it's handy to have some equipment. Here are some tools that can be used to progress beyond your bodyweight. Some of these you can take with you and others can be stored in your house or car:

- Resistance bands
- Light/medium weight dumb bells
- Inflatable Swiss balls (the small ones)
- A pull up/ dip station (If you have the money) This is a very handy station which has multiple uses and exercises you can do. Mainly pull ups and Dips.
- Yoga mat
- Meditation or relaxation music tapes handy (help reduce stress)
- Resistance Bands (to increase muscle strength and use for upper body pulling exercises.

IMPORTANT NOTE: Buyer Beware!

There are some exercise aids that have been specifically marketed to walkers – things like weighted shoes to add resistance while jogging or brisk-walking. Before you dole out your cash to buy exercise accessories, speak to a fitness trainer or orthopedist first. Some products can be just commercial hype. This article on www.walking.about.com can shed some light on the subject.

The same goes for a lot of those abdominal infomercials which are heavily marketed and promise six pack abs! If it sounds too good to be true it probably is!

If you're going cross-country driving and the trip will take many hours, schedule hourly stops so you can perform some stretching exercises, or go for a 15-minute walk. Exercising will energize you, diminishing your need for frequent cups of coffee and relieve eye strain.

How to Make Your Own Strap Suspension Trainer

If you'll be working out at home or have little access to equipment, the problem always lies in the pulling exercises. Resistance training is dependent on gravity. Without access to big machines to redirect resistance or barbells and dumbbells to use, you'll need to make use of your own body weight. This is another alternative or a good addition to light weight resistance bands.

Again, because resistance training is dependent on gravity, you have to orient your body in line with it in order to stress your muscles. That means something like a pull up bar that we listed above. If you don't have a pull up bar or a place to put one, you can easily construct an apparatus called a suspension trainer. Let's go over how you can do this easily.

There are a few strap suspension devices on the market for upwards of $150-$200. You don't need to spend anywhere near that amount. We'll show you how to make your own that is equally as effective for a lot less money that you can use at home. This isn't the best exercise device in the world, but can be crucial if you don't have access to some kind of pulling exercise device. Here's how you do it.

1. Go to Amazon www.amazon.com and pick up the pair of Body Solid NB59 Adjustable Nylon Cable Handles. Also pick up 2 small Black Diamond Neutrino carabiners.

2. Go to this link at Strapworks www.strapworks.com and pick up 20 ft. of Tubular Nylon Webbing.

3. From here it is simple. In each end of the webbing, tie an overhand know to form a loop. Connect your carabiner. And attach to the exercise handle. Tie a knot mid-strap to use as a door anchor.

This device will then allow you to anchor to some stable object or over top of a door frame by tying a knot in then end opposite the handles. You can adjust the length of how long each handle is either by putting the carabiner in a lower or higher D-ring or by tying the anchoring knot farther up or down the webbing.

Depending on how you stand and at what angle your body is at, will determine how much of your body weight you'll be using. Over time, you can make your exercise progressive by using more of your body weight. Eventually progressing all the way up to your own body weight for multiple pull ups or chin ups. You now have a simple homemade device to assist in your upper body pulling movements among other areas. Whole routines have been designed around this simple device. Without going into all of the funky training moves, just use this device to replace the conventional exercises you may not have the current piece of equipment for (chest press, rows, bicep curl).

Hotels

Back to the hotel scene: Most hotels have gyms you can use free of charge. Get up early and make time to get some exercise in before you get too busy with meetings.

Nice hotels have spa facilities that you can enjoy while on a business trip. Reward yourself with a massage AFTER an intense training session which will help loosen up the tired muscles and possibly aid in recovery.

If you can't make the gym or would rather workout in peace then do some bodyweight training in the hotel room using the principles and exercises listed above.

Alternatively, if there is a sport you like playing see if there are any activities in the hotel for your chosen sport.

A good motivator, or exercise aid, is to invest in a good mp3 or I-pod. Make a playlist with some motivating music that helps get you moving. Or you could go to you tube and get motivating.

Always Carry

Always have the following items with you as you travel:

- Comfortable shoes
- Padlock
- Foldable, light gym bag
- Quick dry clothing
- Resistance bands
- An MP3 or music device

You can keep these in your suitcase at all times so you don't waste time looking for them and re-packing them. A busy individual like you need not be unencumbered by exercise paraphernalia that you're hunting for just before taking a flight!

Keep a Diary!

Keeping a workout diary or progress chart is a good way to track your progress with your program. One of the keys to changing your body is to make sure you are progressing in one way or another.

Write down the reps you perform for each exercise, then on your next workout try to go one better and increase your reps or weight as often as possible going forward.

This also helps keep you motivated as you can see your improvements day to day. The reason people reach plateaus in their training is because they don't change the weight or give their body a different stimulus.

Progressive overload is one of the main principles of resistance training. Simply stated: It means you subject the body to a greater stress than what it's accustomed to in a process over time.

A workout sheet like the one below is available to download just click on the chart.

84

S.P.A.R.T.A.
Sports Performance And Resistance Training Association

Name: _____

Phone: _____

Goals: _____

Exercises/Settings:	Date: Weight:									

Notes

Measure Date: _____ Arm: _____ Chest: _____ Waist: _____ Hip: _____ Thigh: _____ Body Fat: ___ ___ ___ = _____ = _____%

SECTION 5: INFORMATION/RESOURCES FOR THE BUSY PERSON

There are some handy free resources you can use here to help you on your quest for a healthier lifestyle.

This website http://www.exrx.net/index.html is free and has over 1400 exercises, some fitness assessments and calculators and more information on nutrition.

Here are some others:

- Visit my blog: http://www.specialisedpersonaltraining.com which I update with articles on exercise and nutrition
- www.myfitnesspal.com – This is a handy website and also an app you can download on your phone to track calories
- http://www.exrx.net/index.html – Exercise instructions and Visual Demonstrations
- www.fitday.com – Online diet journal
- www.fitbusinessman.com – Free resources and articles for the busy professional

My friend, Chris Lutz, wrote a very comprehensive book on high intensity metabolic training. This can be bought on **Amazon here**.

Fitness-Friendly Hotels

Suzanne Schlosberg performed some helpful due diligence to help the busy traveler by providing the names of major hotels with gym facilities (US only). An extract from that list:

Four Seasons – 95% of their hotels have pools. All of their fitness centers have cardio and weight machines;

Ritz Carlton – 80% of their hotels have pools
Sheraton Hotels and Resorts – pool facility in 95% of their hotels

Westin Hotels and Resorts, all of their hotels have pools.[2]

Fitness-Friendly Airports

There are some airports that have gyms also. For a list from the US and Canada visit this website: http://airportgyms.com/mobile/

If you are looking for something more relaxing, here are a couple of airports that have massage facilities:

Chicago: O'Hare International Airport – *A Massage Inc*, level 6, main terminal west (near post office); open 7:30 am to 9:30 pm

Boston: Logan International Airport – *A Relaxed Attitude* – terminal B, American Airlines Side, upper level (hours vary);

Seattle: Seattle-Tacoma International Airport – *Massage Bar Inc.* – Concourse C, beyond security checkpoint, Gates N-16 and N-1

CONCLUSION

When you started reading this book, you probably didn't think you could ever incorporate a fitness program into your busy lifestyle. Now, however, you should feel empowered and ready to start your fitness regime!

Remember some of the rules we covered here. You can go back and re-read different sections at any time.

Let's just highlight a few of the most important principles that you should bear in mind as you move forward:

Start off slow and then progress from there, don't go from not working out to doing 6 days a week!

Exercise for *more* than your look, your body needs to be fit and healthy if you want to live a disease free life.

Always plan ahead with exercise and nutrition – Fail to plan means planning to fail!

Carry essential fitness tools with you as you travel.

Eat healthy and properly so that you have energy to workout.

Keep a workout log with your progress.

Exercise with friends or other people who share a common fitness interest with you (and make NEW friends in the process!)

Manage your time effectively so that you can incorporate a fitness program – large or small – into your daily routine.

Now that you've obtained the information you need, the next step is up to you. If you lack motivation then hiring a Personal Trainer can be useful. But here you have a plan that will keep you in good shape. Consult the resources recommended in this book, including the websites, and build an exercise program into your life.

What will your rewards be for your efforts? Statistically, you'll:

Look better
Feel better
Be more productive
Have a higher quality of life

And, in case it matters to you..

You'll be also be the envy of your busy colleagues and friends who will be asking you how you do it!

GOOD LUCK AND GET MOVING!

ABOUT THE AUTHOR

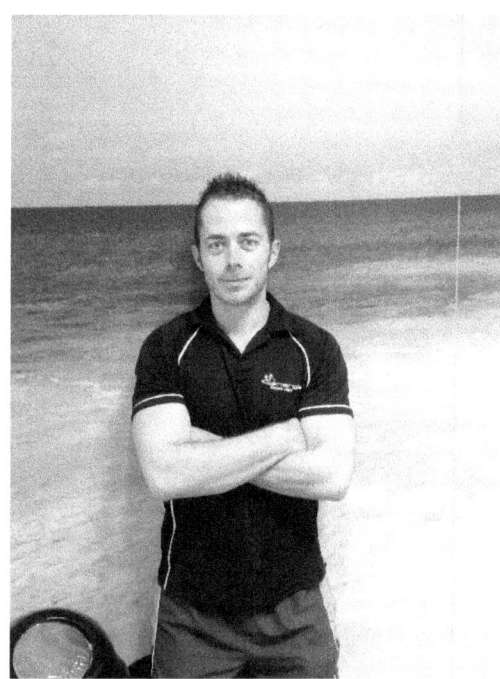

Nigel is an experienced personal trainer from Ireland and works in Dublin where he operates as an independent personal trainer.

Nigel has a passion for helping people from all walks of life and all over the world achieve their goals. He uses a science based exercise program to give his clients safe, effective and time efficient workouts.

Among his many achievements are helping one of his clients lose over 60 lbs. in 8 months. He has done presentations all over the world and locally on a broad range of topics regarding exercise and nutrition. He also operates a blog where he writes about proper exercise methodology.

He specialises in higher intensity, shorter duration workouts for busy professionals.

He believes people can achieve a great physique without being a slave to the gym. Nigel also has qualifications in the field of personal training and fitness, health studies and a degree in business.

You can find out more and read articles by Nigel at www.specialisedpersonaltraining.com